Bahy Ahmed Ali

Hepatitis B Virus (HBV) and Its Vertical Transmission

Bahy Ahmed Ali

Hepatitis B Virus (HBV) and Its Vertical Transmission

LAP LAMBERT Academic Publishing

Impressum / Imprint

Bibliografische Information der Deutschen Nationalbibliothek: Die Deutsche Nationalbibliothek verzeichnet diese Publikation in der Deutschen Nationalbibliografie; detaillierte bibliografische Daten sind im Internet über http://dnb.d-nb.de abrufbar.

Alle in diesem Buch genannten Marken und Produktnamen unterliegen warenzeichen-, marken- oder patentrechtlichem Schutz bzw. sind Warenzeichen oder eingetragene Warenzeichen der jeweiligen Inhaber. Die Wiedergabe von Marken, Produktnamen, Gebrauchsnamen, Handelsnamen, Warenbezeichnungen u.s.w. in diesem Werk berechtigt auch ohne besondere Kennzeichnung nicht zu der Annahme, dass solche Namen im Sinne der Warenzeichen- und Markenschutzgesetzgebung als frei zu betrachten wären und daher von jedermann benutzt werden dürften.

Bibliographic information published by the Deutsche Nationalbibliothek: The Deutsche Nationalbibliothek lists this publication in the Deutsche Nationalbibliografie; detailed bibliographic data are available in the Internet at http://dnb.d-nb.de.

Any brand names and product names mentioned in this book are subject to trademark, brand or patent protection and are trademarks or registered trademarks of their respective holders. The use of brand names, product names, common names, trade names, product descriptions etc. even without a particular marking in this work is in no way to be construed to mean that such names may be regarded as unrestricted in respect of trademark and brand protection legislation and could thus be used by anyone.

Coverbild / Cover image: www.ingimage.com

Verlag / Publisher:
LAP LAMBERT Academic Publishing
ist ein Imprint der / is a trademark of
OmniScriptum GmbH & Co. KG
Heinrich-Böcking-Str. 6-8, 66121 Saarbrücken, Deutschland / Germany
Email: info@lap-publishing.com

Herstellung: siehe letzte Seite /
Printed at: see last page
ISBN: 978-3-659-71140-4

Contents

Introduction

The Hepatitis B virus (HBV) is a mostly double-stranded DNA virus in the Hepadnaviridae family. HBV is a common viral pathogen that causes a substantial health burden worldwide. Significant progress has been made in the past few decades in understanding the natural history of HBV infection (**Pungpapong et al., 2007**). One of five hepatitis viruses, HBV causes acute and chronic hepatitis in humans. Despite the current availability of an effective vaccine, almost 1.2 million people worldwide still die each year from HBV related diseases (Center for Disease Control **CDC**). An acute HBV infection usually causes only mild symptoms and the majority of infected adults successfully clear the virus and acquires life-long immunity. In acute hepatitis, it takes about 1 to 6 months from the time of infection for the disease to manifest itself. Early symptoms include nausea and vomiting, loss of appetite, fatigue, and muscle and joint aches. Jaundice, together with dark urine and light stools, follows. Only about 1 percent of patients infected with hepatitis B die due to liver damage in this early stage. The risk of becoming chronically infected depends on the age at the time of infection. More than 90 percent of newborns, 50 percent of children, 5 percent of adults infected with HBV develop chronic hepatitis. Those who are unable to produce an effective immune response allow the virus to replicate for long periods in their livers, causing chronic hepatitis HBV infection, cirrhosis of the liver, and hepatocellular carcinoma (HCC) (**Yen, 2002**). Transmission of the hepatitis B virus is through contact with blood and other bodily fluid. Chronic hepatitis B is treated with a manufactured form of interferon, a protein made naturally by the body to boost the immune system and to regulate other cell functions (**CDC**). A vaccine is available to prevent HBV which originally consisted of purified HBV surface antigens (HBsAg) prepared from the serum of carriers and wash chemically treated to kill any contaminating viruses, but the current vaccine is genetically engineered HBsAg produced in yeasts ((**Yen, 2002**).

A dynamic balance between viral replication and host immune response is pivotal to the pathogenesis of liver disease. In immune-competent adults, most HBV infections spontaneously resolve, whereas in most neonates and infants they become chronic. Those with chronic HBV may present in 1 of 4 phases of infection: (1) in a state of immune tolerance, (2) with hepatitis B e antigen (HBeAg)–positive chronic hepatitis, (3) as an inactive hepatitis B surface antigen carrier, or (4) with HBeAg negative chronic hepatitis. Of these, HBeAg-positive and HBeAg-negative chronic hepatitis may progress to cirrhosis and its long term sequelae including hepatic decompensation and hepatocellular carcinoma. Several prognostic factors, such as serum HBV DNA concentrations, HBeAg status, serum aminotransferases, and certain HBV genotypes, have been identified to predict long-term outcome. These data emphasize the importance of monitoring all patients with chronic HBV infection to identify candidates for and select optimal timing of antiviral treatment, to recognize those at risk of complications, and to implement surveillance for early detection of hepatocellular carcinoma (**Pungpapong** *et al.*, **2007**).

HBV enters the body through direct blood exposure and through sexual contact. Fewer than 5% of adults infected with HBV become carriers and remain infected with HBV for longer than six months. For people who are infected with HBV at birth or as young children, the risk of becoming a carrier may be as high as 90%. An estimated 350 million people worldwide are chronically infected with HBV, 25% of whom develop serious liver damage. HBV is responsible for up to 80% of all cases of liver cancer worldwide. In **2006**, the U.S. Centers for Disease Control and Prevention (CDC) estimated that 46,000 Americans were newly infected with HBV and between 1-1.4 million persons have chronic HBV infection. Health Canada estimates that 5,000 or more people in Canada are newly infected with HBV each year, and that 240,000 Canadians are chronically infected. Asians and immigrants from other areas of the world where hepatitis B is endemic have higher rates of infection; most are infected at birth or as young children. Most people infected with HBV do not have symptoms and lead normal lives. However, in about 25% of cases HBV can cause

4

serious liver damage – including fibrosis and cirrhosis – usually over several years or decades. In severe cases, hepatitis B can lead to liver failure and death. An effective vaccine is available to prevent HBV. There are also various treatments that can help slow or stop disease progression.

Clements *et al.*, **(2010)** raise the possibility of a threat to the global hepatitis B immunization programme because of the use of lamivudine and other nucleoside or nucleotide analogue therapeutic agents to treat individuals with chronic hepatitis B infection. Although the threat is theoretical, there is already evidence that current treatment regimens have resulted in the selection of stable ADAP-VEMs. Even though the transmission of ADAP-VEMs to individuals immunized with HBV vaccine has been observed in only one case (**Thibault** *et al.*, **2002**), VEMs generated by HB vaccine have spread more widely and caused infection in previously immunized individuals.

Knowing this, what should our response be now? At the very least, we must learn more about ADAP-VEMs, their transmissibility and their potential to cause infection and disease in immunized individuals. This will require virological surveillance and clinical follow-up of infected individuals and those undergoing treatment, and also, possibly, surveillance of their close contacts. The initial focus of these activities should be high-risk settings until the level of risk is defined and understood better. Incident cases of HBV in these situations could also be examined for VEMs, especially if a new case is epidemiologically linked to an individual undergoing treatment for chronic hepatitis B infection. Follow-up of such cases of HBV, however, would depend on the availability of testing, and currently no suitable commercial tests are available.

At present, treatment aims to prevent the long-term complications of HBV infection, with little consideration given to potential adverse public health impacts. The number of potent antiviral agents is limited, their development by manufacturers is episodic and trials that have evaluated combination therapies are lacking. Because of these factors, monotherapy remains the usual practice in most settings. As with other infections, more potent combination therapies for HBV would reduce the chance of drug-resistance and lead to early and longer-lasting control of HBV replication. Such therapies would not only benefit the individual but would also simultaneously reduce the likelihood that ADAP-VEMs of global public health significance will emerge. Trials are urgently needed to identify the optimal combination of existing drugs that can address both individual and public health needs. International therapeutic guidelines for chronic HB such as those issued by the Asian-Pacific Association for the Study of the Liver (**Liaw *et al.*, 2008**), the European Association for the Study of the Liver International Consensus Conference and the American Association for the Study of Liver Disease (**Lok and McMahon, 2008**) should ideally consider both of these elements, and will need to be refined as more is learned about ADAP-VEMs. More effective novel agents are clearly needed that target other parts of the virus.

It is still essential to prevent the spread of wild, vaccine-sensitive strains of HBV. Well-tested measures such as safe sex and avoiding the risks associated with injection drug use will also help to reduce horizontal transmission of both the wild virus and VEMs. HB immunization for infants of mothers with HBV will reduce perinatal transmission of the wild virus but may not prevent transmission of VEMs. The global HB immunization programme will continue to reduce new incident infections of hepatitis B and the burden of chronic HBV disease globally, although it is simultaneously generating VEMs.

Globally

- Estimated 2 billion people infected with HBV.

- 400 million have chronic HBV infection

- Approximately 88% of the world's population live in areas where the prevalence of chronic HBV infection is high (>8% HBsAg +) or moderate (2-7% HBsAg +).

- About 1.2 million people worldwide still die each year from HBV related diseases (Center for Disease Control **CDC**)

- The **CDC** estimates that 1-1.4 million Americans are chronically infected with HBV, but other researchers suggest that, when undocumented immigrants and others are considered, the number is closer to 2 million.

- An estimated 2,000-4,000 Americans die each year due to complications related to HB.

- Health Canada estimates that 240,000 Canadians are chronically infected with HBV.

- Immigrants from Asia, the Middle East, and parts of Africa—and their children—are at higher risk for HBV infection (**Figure 1**).

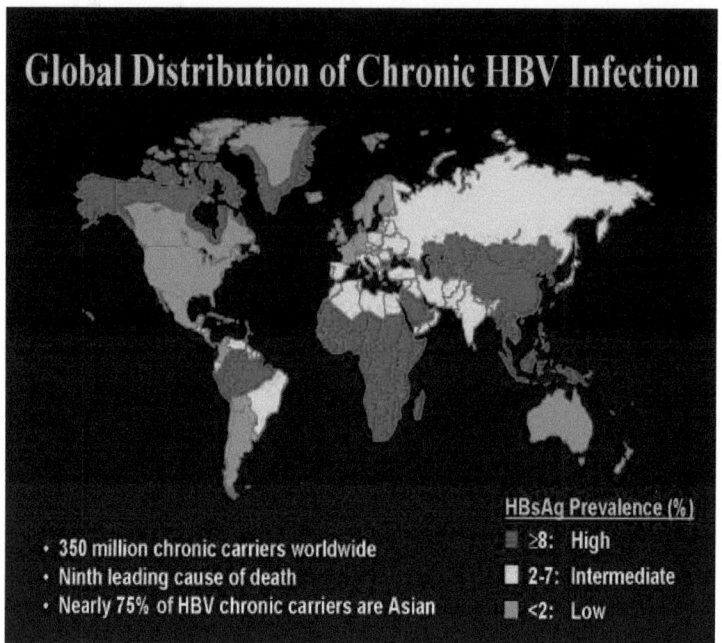

Global Distribution of Chronic HBV Infection

· 350 million chronic carriers worldwide
· Ninth leading cause of death
· Nearly 75% of HBV chronic carriers are Asian

HBsAg Prevalence (%)
■ ≥8: High
■ 2-7: Intermediate
■ <2: Low

Figure (1): Global Distribution of Chronic HBV Infection: The prevalence of chronic HBV infection is low (<2%) in the general population in Northern and Western Europe, North America, Australia, New Zealand, Mexico, and southern South America (Map 2-2). The prevalence of chronic HBV infection is intermediate (2%–7%) in South, Central, and Southwest Asia, Israel, Japan, Eastern and Southern Europe, Russia, most areas surrounding the Amazon River basin, Honduras, and Guatemala (see Map 2-2). The prevalence of chronic HBV infection is high (≥8%) in all socioeconomic groups in: all of Africa; Southeast Asia, including China, Korea, Indonesia, and the Philippines; the Middle East, except Israel; South and Western Pacific islands; the interior Amazon River basin; and certain parts of the Caribbean (Haiti and the Dominican Republic) (see Map 2-2). **Chaves (2010)**

Universal HB vaccination is recommended by the World Health Organization; today, teenagers are routinely vaccinated against HBV, but infant vaccination is still optional in several states. The American Academy of Pediatrics recommends HBV vaccination for all infants.

HBV Genome and Genotypes

The HBV virion genome is circular and approximately 3.2 kb in size and consists of DNA that is mostly double stranded. It has compact organization, with four overlapping reading frames running in one direction and no noncoding regions. The minus strand is unit length and has a protein covalently attached to the 5' end. The other strand, the plus strand, is variable in length, but has less than unit length, and has an RNA oligonucleotide at its 5' end. The four genes encoded are core (pre-core and core proteins), surface (pre-Sl, pre-S2 and S proteins), X and polymerase (**Figure 2**). The core gene encodes the core nucleocapsid protein and the secreted, soluble hepatitis Be antigen (HBeAg) protein. The surface gene encodes pre-Sl, pre-S2 and S protein, yielding the large-, middle- and small-surface proteins, respectively. The X gene encodes the X protein, which has transactivating properties and may be important in hepatic carcinogenesis. The polymerase gene encodes a large protein with functions critical for DNA replication and packaging (**Bartholomeusz _et al._, 2003**).

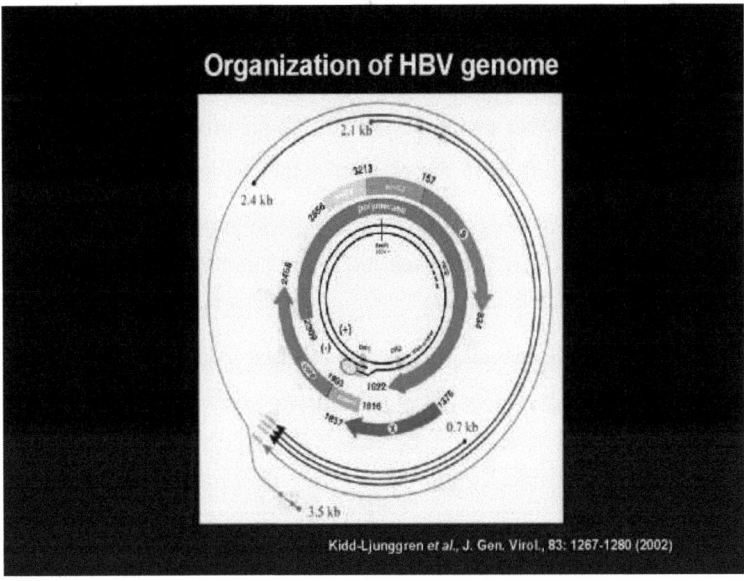

Organization of HBV genome

Kidd-Ljunggren et al., J. Gen. Virol., 83: 1267-1280 (2002)

Figure (2): HBV Genome

Genotypes or genetic subtypes describe genetically related strains and have been described for viruses belonging to several different families. The eight major genotypes of HB virus (HBV) have distinct geographic distribution. Recent studies suggest possible pathogenic and therapeutic differences among HBV genotypes. HBV has been classified into eight genotypes from A to H (**Idrees *et al.*, 2004**); and four major serotypes, *ayw, ayr, adw* and *adr*, on the basis of complete genome and S gene sequence analysis (**Arauz-Ruiz *et al.*, 2002**).

A sequence divergence of 8% or greater has been observed in the entire genome sequences (**Sakurai *et al.*, 2004**). The genotypes of HBV have distinct geographical distributions, which have been associated with anthropologic history (**Orito *et al.*, 2001a,b**). Genotypes and serotypes are useful tools for understanding the epidemiology of HBV infection. Although both genotypes and serotypes segregate geographically (**Table 1**), the same serotype can be represented by several genotypes (**Arankalle *et al.*, 2003**).

Recently, genotypes of HBV have been reported to be an influential factor in the clinical manifestations of chronic liver disease in the host. Genotype A is associated with chronic liver disease more frequently than genotype D in Europe Genotype C induces more severe liver disease than genotype B found in Asia (**Kao *et al.*, 2000**). Furthermore, it was reported that genotype B had two subgroups (**Sugauchi *et al.*, 2002**), and these subgroups influence the clinical manifestations of liver disease in these patients. Restriction fragment length polymorphism (RFLP) of polymerase chain reaction (PCR) products has been used for genotyping hepatitis C, but for HB, it has been used only to relate restriction patterns to serotypes. Only three reports have been published from India; all of them show that genotype D is the most common genotype among Indian population (**Arankalle *et al.*, 2003; Gandhe *et al.*, 2003**).

Table (1): HBV genotypes, subtypes and their distribution

Genotype	Serotype	Distribution
A	*Adw2,ayw1*	North-West Europe, United States, sub-Saharan Africa, Central and South America
B	*Adw2,ayw*	East Asia, south east Asia
C	*Adw2,adrq+,adrq-,ayr,adr*	East Asia, south east Asia, pacific islands
D	*Ayw2,ayw3,ayw4*	Mediterranean and central Europe, Middle East, Central Asia, India, South America
E	*Awy4*	West Africa, southern Africa
F	*Adw4q-,adw2,adw4*	Central America, south America, Polynesia
G	*Adw2*	United states of America, France (and still to be determined(
H	*Adw4*	Central America

In a country like Egypt, where **more than 4.7 million people** are estimated to be infected with HBV, it is useful to discriminate between sporadic and endemic HBV infections. In Egypt, few reports described the frequency of HBV genotypes in Egypt. In previous study, genotype D was reported as the predominant HBV genotype in the study subjects (37.1%) followed by genotype B that constituted 25.7%. These figures are in conformity with 2 other studies done in Egypt. In one study, the genotypes of HBV isolated from 105 serum samples from Egyptian carriers were determined by sequencing and found that HBV genotype D are most prevalent in Egypt (**Saudy *et al.*, 2003**). This study is in conformity with 2 other studies done in Egypt. In one study, the genotypes of HBV isolated from 105 serum samples from Egyptian carriers were determined by sequencing and found that HBV genotype D are most prevalent in Egypt. Examined 2 serum samples positive for HBV DNA by primer specific PCR and these turned to be of genotype D but they didn't find other genotypes as they only examined 2 serum samples for hepatitis B virus corresponding to six major genotypes by PCR using type-specific primers.

A recent study carried out by **Saudy** *et al.,* **(2003)** observed the prevalence of HBsAg to be 5.7 %, which is similar to that observed from other parts of Egypt. For such a purpose, characteristic markers are used to discriminate between identical or different genotypes and subtypes in a population. Another study showed that HBV infections in randomly Egyptian patients' are attributed predominantly to viral genotypes D and C that constituted 57.5% and 22.5%, respectively of the total infections. In addition, there was a relatively prevalence of other HBV genotypes such as E and F that constituted 15 % and 5 % respectively for each one .on the other hand different HBV subtypes have been detected such as *Ayw* (70%), *Adr*(20%), and *Adw* (10%).. No HBV genotype A or B was found in our study and furthermore, genotypes G and H were not determined (**Mogahed, 2009**).

The subtypes in the S region are also useful markers for this purpose. The relationship of the genotype to clinical manifestations and treatment response has also been shown. In the present study the HBV genotypes of 42 samples were determined by RFLP analysis and sequencing of desired regions to determine variations and identify the subtypes of the surface region.

Genotype D was most prevalent. Genotyping was carried out by RFLP analysis and confirmed by sequencing. Nucleotide sequences showed significant homology (96–97%) with the other genotypes that have been reported. Subtype *ayw* was the most prevalent subtype within the surface region. Construction of a phylogenetic tree incorporating these isolates and other published HBV sequences showed that the isolates are derived from the same evolutionary tree. The study adds to our understanding of the genetic diversity of HBV and the geographical distribution of its subtypes, and will be useful for reconstructing the evolutionary history of HBV. This study showed that HBV infections in randomly Egyptian patients' are attributed predominantly to viral genotypes D and C that constituted 57.5% and 22.5%, respectively of the total infections. In addition, there was a relatively prevalence of other HBV genotypes such as E and F that constituted 15 % and 5 % respectively for each one .on the other hand different HBV subtypes have been detected such as *Ayw* (70%), *Adr* (20%), and *Adw* (10%).. No HBV genotype A or B was found in our study and furthermore, genotypes G and H were not determined.

HBV Replication

The virus in the serum adheres to the surface of the hepatocytes through a receptor. Through the process of endocytosis the virus enters the cell and is uncoated to remove the envelope proteins. The viral core particles bind to the nuclear pore and the HBV genome enters the nucleus. In the nucleus the HBV DNA is repaired and chromatinized to form a mini-chromosome. The mini-chromosome is used as the transcriptional template for RNA synthesis by RNA Polymerase II. The HBV RNA is transported into the cytoplasm where the viral proteins are made. The pre-genomic RNA is encapsulated. In the viral RNA cores DNA synthesis occurs through a process of reverse transcription and also DNA synthesis. The viral cores can be either transported back into the nucleus for further genomic amplification, or are enveloped and secreted into the blood (**Figure 3**).

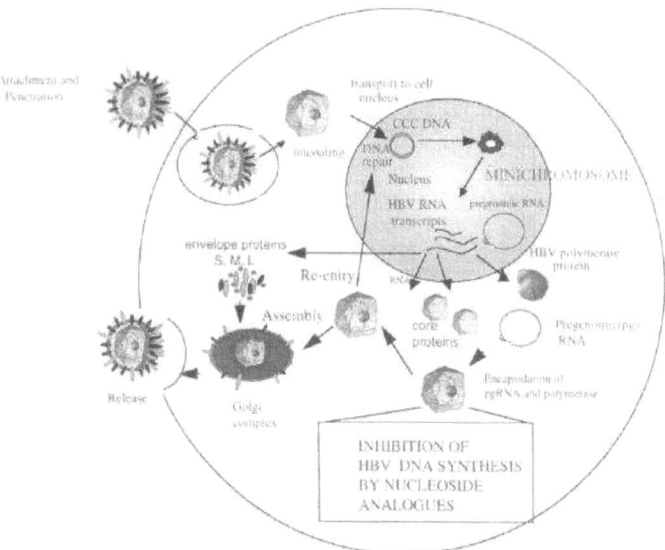

Figure (3). Hepatitis B virus replication cycle

HB Antigens:

There are three different types of hepatitis b antigens encoded by the HBV genome.

- HB Surface antigen (Hbsag)- There are three different types of hepatitis B surface antigens; small hepatitis B surface antigen (Hbsag or SHBsAg), middle hepatitis B surface antigen (MHBsAg), and large hepatitis B surface Antigen (LHBsAg). HBsAg is the smallest protein of the hepatitis B surface proteins and has historically been known as the Australia antigen (Au antigen). It is very hydrophobic, containing four-transmembrane spanning regions. This protein is the prime constituent of all hepatitis b particle forms and appears to be manufactured by the virus in high quantities. It also contains a highly antigenic epitope which may be responsible for triggering immune response. Regardless of the high antigeniticy and prevalence of these particles, the immune system appears basically oblivious to their presence. Reduced production of HBsAg leads to intracellular retention of the virus. MHBsAg contains an additional amino-acid domain and appears to reside extracellularly. Although some believe that the MHBsAg is responsible for HBV attachment, MHBsAg is not required for HBV infectivity and therefore it is more likely that is contributes to viral attachment as a secondary mechanism. LHBsAg is the largest of the HBV surface proteins, containing three domains within the HBV encoding region. HBV is believed to be involved in liver attachment due to its variability among patients. It is also believed to be responsible for mediating viral attachment into host cells, although this has yet to be confirmed experimentally.

- HB Core Antigen (HBcAg)- The only HBV antigen that cannot be detected directly by blood test, this antigen can only be isolated by analyzing an infected hepatocyte. A 185 amino acid protein is expressed in the cytoplasm of infected cells; they are highly associated with nucleocapsid assembly.

- HB e Antigen (HBeAg)- The e antigen is named due to its "early" appearance during an acute HBV infection. Thought to be located in the core structure of the virus molecule, this antigen can be detected by blood test. If found its usually indicative of complete virus particles in circulation **(Yen, 2002)**.

HBV Transmission

HBV is transmitted by direct blood-to-blood contact. A major transmission route is sharing drug equipment for both injection and non-injection drugs (including needles, cookers, tourniquets, cocaine straws, and crack pipes). Needles used for tattooing and body piercing may also spread the virus. Sharing personal items such as razors, toothbrushes, and nail files is a less likely but still possible transmission route. This can happen when a small amount of HBV-infected blood remains on an item after use and is transferred to another person who uses the same item.

In the past, many people contracted HBV through blood transfusions; however, a test for HBV in donated blood has been in use since 1972 and a test for HCV became available in 1992. Today, blood transfusions are considered safe. Health-care workers may be exposed to HBV through needle-sticks and other accidental exposures on the job. HBV is present in semen and vaginal fluids, and HB may be transmitted through sexual activity. HBV is much more likely than HCV to be sexually transmitted. The **CDC** estimates that the majority of new HBV infections in the United States may be sexually transmitted. Transmission may be more likely during a woman's menstrual period. HBV transmission rates are particularly high among men who have sex with men.

Perinatal transmission from HBV-infected mothers to their infants before or during birth account for the majority of infections in areas where HBV is endemic. Transmission is more likely if the mother has a high level of HBV in her blood; mothers coinfected with HCV or HIV in addition to HBV also appear to be more likely to transmit hepatitis B to their babies. Although HB surface antigen, a particle of the virus, is present in breast milk, there is no evidence that hepatitis B is transmitted through breast-feeding if the infant is vaccinated (**Figure 4**).

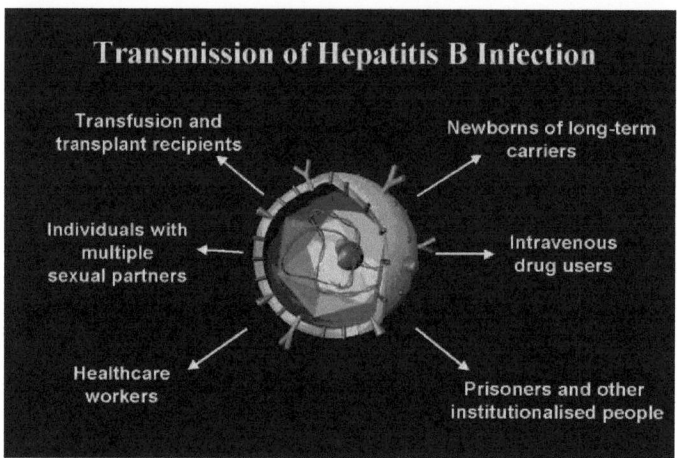

Figure (4): Transmission of HB Infection

Studies indicate that HBV transmission is common between young children in areas where the virus is endemic, probably due to scratching and biting. Although HBV is detectable in saliva, HB is not known to be transmitted by sneezing, coughing, or sharing eating utensils or drinking glasses; household transmission of HBV rarely occurs. There are no documented cases of HBV transmission through urine, feces, sweat, tears, or vomit. In one-third or more cases, people have no identifiable risk factors and the route of hepatitis B transmission is unknown (**Sookoian, 2006**).

Vertical Transmission of HBV

Vertical transmission of HB virus (HBV) is the main cause of chronic HBV infection in endemic areas. When the mother is a chronic HBsAg carrier (and positive for viral DNA in her serum), the risk of the neonates to become a chronic carrier himself is closed to 80 to 90% **(Lee *et al*., 2006)**. In the opposite, if the mother is negative for viral DNA in the serum, the transmission rate is about 10 to 30%. In the case of hepatitis C virus (HCV), the risk of perinatal transmission is approximately 4% to 10%, although reported rates of transmission vary depending on virus genotype, co-infection with human immunodeficiency virus (HIV) and titer of HCV-RNA in the mother **(Tajiri *et al*., 2001)**. Risk is more important if the woman had elevated levels of viral load (> 105 copies/mL) and if the duration between membrane rupture and delivery is long.

There are three possible routes of transmission of hepatitis virus from infected mothers to infants: transplacental transmission in uterus (antenatal transmission), transmission during delivery and postnatal transmission from mothers to infants during child- care or through breast- feeding. In the case of HBV infection, several evidences demonstrate that in uterus infection plays an important role. Besides, most researchers hold that the mechanism of HBV intrauterine infection is transplacental infection. In fact, it was suggested that transplacental leakage of HBeAg-positive maternal blood, which is induced by uterine contractions during pregnancy and the disruption of placental barriers, is the most likely route to cause HBV intrauterine infection. In addition, it was shown that the main risk factors for intrauterine HBV infection are maternal serum HBeAg positivity, history of threatened preterm labor, and HBV in the placenta especially the villous capillary endothelial cells **(Xu *et al*., 2002)**. Therefore, the presence of HBsAg in cord blood may indicate intrauterine infection. Unfortunately, intrauterine transmission of HBV can be a possible cause of vaccination failure and spread of HBV. An interesting finding is the fact that some of the fetuses that have contact with HBV antigens early in embryonic development may become immunologically tolerant to HBV antigens. Finally, in both HBV and HCV chronic infection, high maternal viremia and intrapartum exposure to virus-contaminated maternal blood increased the risk of virus transmission during vaginal deliveries.

> **Vertical Transmission Via Germ Cells**

HBV antigens were detected in human semen, and it is now well-established that this biological fluid is a vector for the spread of hepatitis B. However, few studies have tried to identify the contaminated cells within semen. It has been reported that HBV DNA was integrated into the DNA of spermatozoa in two of three patients with acute hepatitis, suggesting that there may be true transmission of HBV via the germ line. Another study of chronic HBV antigen carriers showed that HBV DNA was present in all of the semen samples tested, with the infected cells being both spermatozoa and mononuclear cells. Persistent free HBV DNA has also been detected in the semen of patients with no markers of viral replication in serum, indicating that the genital tract may act as a reservoir and that these patients may transmit the virus sexually.

The known transmissions of HBV do not constitute a menace to man because we are able to identify effective preventive measures. The unknown transmissions have greater risk potential because we do not fully understand their origin. Thus, exploring the feasibility of HBV vertical transmission from parents to their children via germ lines is an exciting program and of substantial importance. To confirm the feasibility of true vertical transmission of HBV via spermatozoa, we have to answer the following question: Does the replication and expression of HBV genes brought into the oocyte via spermatozoon occur in early embryonic cells? However, such studies have been hampered since neither experimental animal nor cell culture systems have been available. The study on replication and expression of HBVDNA in the human embryo would be an ideal model but such a system presents major logistical, moral, and ethical problems. Thus it is crucial to establish a model system for such study. Interspecies in vitro fertilization between human sperm and zona-free hamster ova made it possible. To our knowledge, this is the first time that the IVF technique has been used to study the HBV expression in one- and two-cell embryos originated from golden hamster ova fertilized with human spermatozoa.

Our previous studies have provided the first direct evidence that the HB X, S, C and P genes could be expressed in one- and two-cell embryos originated from golden hamster ova *in vitro* fertilized with human spermatozoa (**Ali et al., 2005; 2006a,b; 2009) (please see Figures 5;6;7; and 8)**. In our studies, we demonstrated that the HBV genes were integrated into the sperm genome and introduced into the zygote of a normal oocyte via IVF with spermatozoon. The sperm-mediated HBV genes also are able to be expressed in early embryonic cells. It may well have farreaching implications for not only human health but also genome reshaping evolutionary processes.

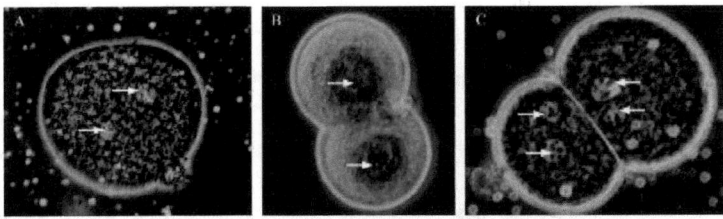

Figure (5): Morphology of normal and abnormal embryos at 24 h after insemination. (A): Normal one-cell embryo showing the male and, female pronuclei (arrows). (B): Normal two-cell embryo showing a nucleus (arrows). in each. (C): Abnormal two-cell embryo showing multiple nuclei in each (arrows).

Using the full-length HBV DNA as a probe, FISH analysis showed a positive signal on the chromosomes of two-cell embryos (**Figure 6**). It provided direct evidence that HBV DNA was integrated into the host genome.

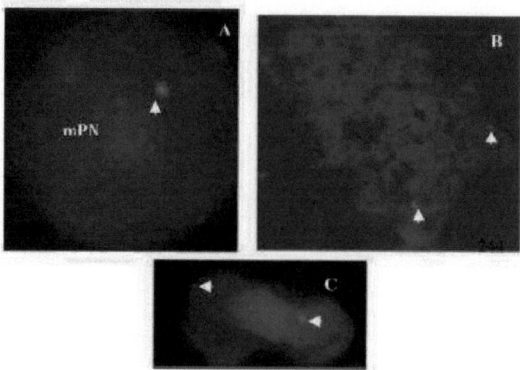

Figure (6). Fluorescence in situ hybridization (FISH) results. Showing clear signals of HBV DNA integrated into (A) the male pronucleus (mPN) and (B) the chromosomes of one-cell embryo, and (C) each nucleus of two-cell embryo (arrows). 1,000 X.

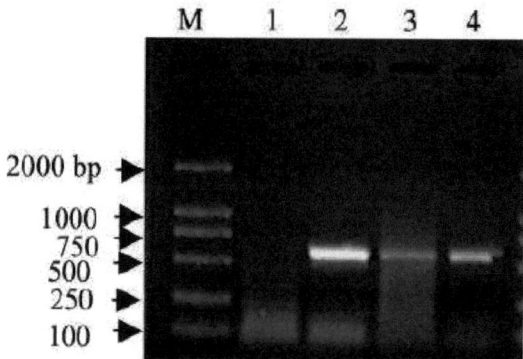

Figure (7). PCR product of HBx gene: lane M, DNA marker (DL2,000); lane 1, negative control; lane 2, positive control; lane 3, one-cell; and lane 4, two-cell embryos. Note: water and pBR322-HBV DNA were used as template in negative and positive control, respectively.

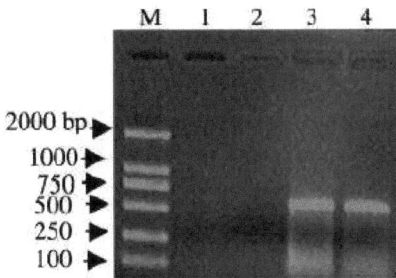

Figure (8). 3. RT-PCR product of HBx gene: lane M, DNA marker (DL2,000); lane 1,minus template control (_T); lane 2,minus reverse transcriptase control (_RT); lane 3, one-cell; and lane 4, two-cell embryos. Note: RT-PCR was carried out using single embryo. Note: The minus template (_T) PCR should have all the PCR components, with water substituted for the RT reaction aliquot. Minus reverse transcriptase control (_RT) containing all the RT reagents except the MMLV Reverse transcriptase.

It can be concluded that the HBV DNA sequences could be brought into the embryo when spermatozoa with integrated HBV DNA penetrated into normal oocytes. The replication and expression of such HBV DNA sequences could occur in early embryonic cells. This *in vitro* culture system bringing HBV DNA into zona-free hamster oocytes via human spermatozoa might be used as a model system for study on the mechanism of true vertical transmission of HBV and hepatotropism. As a whole, the results in this work support the conclusion that human sperm cells can act as vectors for the vertical transmission of HBV genes to the progeny.

➤ **Risk Factors for Vertical Transmission of HBV**

The main risk factor for vertical transmission of HBV seems to be mother viral load. Accordingly, maternal HBV-DNA seems to be a stronger independent predictor of persistent infection than HBeAg status. In effect, vertical transmission was most frequently seen in HBeAg-positive mothers with very high levels of viremia **(Soderstrom *et al.*, 2003)**. Additionally, it was reported that among HBeAg-negative mothers, the Odds Ratio for having a persistently infected infant was 19.2 (95% confidence interval, 2.3- 176.6) in mothers with high versus low levels of serum

HBV-DNA.16 Thus, perinatal exposure to high levels of maternal HBV-DNA is the most important determinant of infection outcome in the infant. On the other hand, it was suggested that the outcome of HBV infection in newborns depends not only on the host's immunocompetence and on viremia level in maternal blood, but also on heterogeneity of HBV. Transmission of mixed HBV populations appears associated with an early immunoelimination of the virus, while infection with wild-type HBV alone contributes to induction of chronicity. Specific allelic mutations in maternal HBV and level of maternal viremia are potential predictors of vertical breakthrough infection.

> **Recommendations to decrease vertical transmission rates**

1- *HBsAg screening* Testing for the hepatitis B virus (HBsAg) is generally a standard, routine test performed on all pregnant women at or before her first pregnancy visit (usually before about 12 to 14 weeks of the pregnancy) **(Mast et al., 2005)**.

2- *Management of infants born to women who are HBsAg positive* An unvaccinated baby whose mother is a hepatitis B carrier has up to a 40% chance of becoming infected with the virus during the first 18 months of their life, of which up to 90% can become a long term carrier and be infectious to others, as well as being at risk of liver disease and liver cancer in later life. Therefore, all infants born to HBsAg positive women should receive HB vaccine and HB Immunoglobulin (HBIG) (0.5 mL) ≤ 12 hours of birth, administered at different injection sites **(Wang et al., 2003)**.

3- Just to remember, HBIG provides passively acquired anti-HBs and temporary protection (i.e., 3-6 months) when administered in standard doses. The vaccine series should be completed according to a recommended schedule for infants born to HBsAg positive mothers.

4- The final dose in the vaccine series should not be administered before age 24 weeks (164 days) **(Lee et al., 2006)**.

5- For preterm infants weighing < 2,000 g, the initial vaccine dose (birth dose) should not be counted as part of the vaccine series because of the potentially reduced immunogenicity of HB vaccine in these infants; 3 additional doses of vaccine (for a total of 4 doses) should be administered beginning when the infant reaches age 1 month **(Mast *et al.*, 2005)**.

6- The HB vaccination can be delayed more than 24 hours after the baby's birth but definitely needs to be given before the baby is 7 days old.

7- Although not indicated in the manufacturer's package labeling, HBsAg containing combination vaccines may be used for infants aged ≥ 6 weeks born to HBsAg positive mothers to complete the vaccine series after receipt of a birth dose of single-antigen HB vaccine and HBIG **(Mast *et al.*, 2005)**.

8- A recent meta-analysis that evaluated the effects of HB vaccine and immunoglobulin in newborn infants of mothers positive for hepatitis B surface antigen, showed that there was no significant difference between recombinant vaccine and plasma derived vaccine on HB infections (relative risk 1.00, 95% CI 0.70 to 1.42) **(Lee *et al.*, 2006)**. However, more infants who received recombinant vaccine achieved antibody levels to hepatitis surface antigen > 10 IU/L. Unfortunately, failure to postnatal immunoprophylaxis for HB has been reported, and specific allelic mutations in maternal HBV and level of maternal viremia were potential predictors of vertical breakthrough infection. Actually, it seems that S variants emerge or are selected under the immune pressure generated by the host or by administration of HB immune globulin and HB vaccination.

9- Mothers who carry the HB virus are encouraged to breastfeed their babies. However, it is recommended that the baby breastfeeds after the administration of the HBIG but not necessarily before the first hepatitis B vaccination (HBV) **(Wang *et al.*, 2003)**.

10-   As HBV transmission through breast milk has been reported in some studies, several groups disagree and do not recommend breast-feeding on the basis of published data.

11-   Finally, as a general advice, it is recommended to explain the mothers that when breast-feeding she should take good care of her nipples, ensuring proper latch-on and allowing the nipples to dry before covering to avoid cracking or bleeding, having in mind that HBV is commonly passed by blood-to-blood routes.

➢ Antiviral Maternal Therapy and Vertical Transmission of HBV

The fact that vertical transmission of HB virus may occasionally occur despite vaccination of the child has prompted to physicians to treat viremic patients with nucleosides analogues to prevent mother-to-child transmission. As regards, some authors observed that in highly viremic HBsAg positive mothers, reduction of viremia by lamivudine therapy in the last month of pregnancy could be an effective and safe measure to reduce the risk of child vaccination breakthrough **(Su _et al._, 2004)**. Moreover, no side effects were observed neither in the mother nor in the babies, observation that had been made before when studying the safety, pharmacokinetics and antiretroviral activity of lamivudine alone and in combination with zidovudine in pregnant women infected with human HIV-1. Nonetheless, in spite of the optimum maternal therapy and neonatal vaccination above reported with encouraging results in controlling vertical transmission, some other authors affirm that lamivudine therapy might not prevent perinatal transmission **(Kazim _et al._, 2002)**. Finally, some researchers introduced a note of caution concerning the use of lamivudine or any other nucleoside during the first trimester of pregnancy, particularly taking into account the possible lethal effects during the embryogenesis **(Divi _et al._, 2005)**.

HBV Disease

> ➤ **HB Symptoms**

Most people with HBV experience few or no symptoms; in fact, many are unaware that they carry the virus. An estimated 30% of people with acute hepatitis B have no symptoms, and most people with chronic HBV also have few or no symptoms. If they do occur, symptoms of acute hepatitis B may include **fatigue** (unusual, prolonged tiredness), **fever, malaise** (a flulike feeling), **nausea, vomiting, loss of appetite** (anorexia), **abdominal pain or bloating, indigestion, headaches, itching** (pruritus), and **muscle or joint aches**.

Rarely, HBV may be associated with rheumatological problems such as polyarteritis nodosa. Some people with either acute or chronic HB may develop jaundice (yellowing of the skin and whites of the eyes), dark urine, and pale-colored stools, caused by a high level of bilirubin (a pigment) in the body. Some people also develop high levels of certain liver enzymes, especially ALT.

> ➤ **Liver Damage**

In a minority of people with hepatitis B, the disease progresses over years or decades, with increasing liver damage. An estimated 20-30% of people with chronic HBV will develop cirrhosis. In severe cases, a person may experience **liver failure and require a liver transplant**. Liver damage may include:

Inflammation: an immune response to infection or injury characterized by infiltration of white blood cells, swelling, and functional impairment of liver cells. People with liver inflammation may – but do not always – have elevated liver enzyme levels.

Necrosis: the death of liver cells (hepatocytes).

Fibrosis: the development of scar tissue within the liver which, if extensive, may begin to interfere with the smooth flow of blood through the liver.

Cirrhosis: a process in which liver cells are destroyed and replaced with scar tissue. Extensive scar formation can impair the flow of blood through the liver.

Compensated cirrhosis is when the liver is scarred but can still work relatively normally; people with compensated cirrhosis usually exhibit few symptoms. Decompensated cirrhosis is when the liver is so damaged that it cannot function properly. People with decompensated cirrhosis may develop complications such as bleeding varices (ruptured blood vessels in the esophagus, stomach, and the gastrointestinal system), abdominal fluid accumulation (ascites), easy bleeding or bruising, mental impairment (hepatic encephalopathy), and coma.

Hepatocellular carcinoma: a type of liver cancer that may occur in people with chronic hepatitis. Liver cancer typically occurs in people with cirrhosis, but some individuals with hepatitis B who develop liver cancer do not have cirrhosis.

➢ **Acute and Chronic HBV**

After exposure to HBV, the incubation period usually lasts 30-90 days. The initial phase of hepatitis B is called acute infection. Clearance of HBV following an acute infection usually takes 2-12 months, during which time a person may experience fatigue and abdominal tenderness (**Figure 9**).

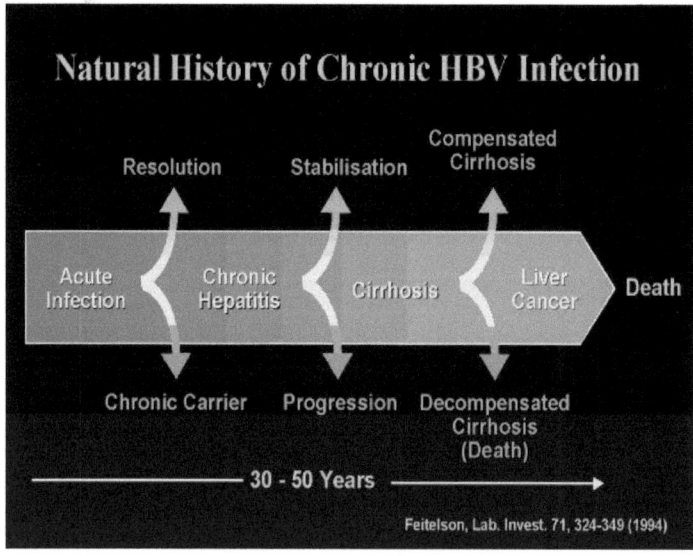

Figure (9): Nature history of Chronic HBV Infection

In a majority of people infected with HBV, the immune system can clear the virus. But some HBV-infected adults – estimated at less than 6% – will become chronically infected, meaning the virus remains in the body after six months. Among people infected with HBV as infants or children, this number is much higher – up to 90% for infants and 30% for children ages 1-5. HBV genetic material (DNA) remains in the nuclei of the cells of everyone infected with the virus, even when HBV infection cannot be detected in the blood. As a result, HBV may reactivate if people's immune systems are damaged or if they receive immunosuppressive drugs such as steroids or chemotherapy. A majority (75%) of people with chronic HB has no symptoms of liver disease, but this situation can change at any time during the life of a carrier.

Those with chronic HBV infection may present: (1) in a state of immune tolerance, (2) with HBeAg-positive chronic hepatitis, (3) as an inactive HBsAg carrier, or (4) with HBeAg-negative chronic hepatitis.

Phase 1

Immune Tolerance

Persistent HBV infection has an initial immune tolerance phase that can be characterized by the presence of HBeAg and high levels of serum HBV DNA due to a high rate of viral replication. This phase is mostly seen in patients who acquire the infection at birth or during early childhood; rarely, it also can be seen briefly in those who acquire the infection in late childhood or adulthood and have subsequent development of chronic HBV infection (**Yim and Lok, 2006**). The absence of liver disease despite high levels of HBV replication is thought to be a consequence of immune tolerance to HBeAg. However, the mechanisms underlying this tolerance are incompletely understood. Experiments in mice suggest that transplacental transfer of maternal HBeAg may induce specific unresponsiveness of T cells to HBeAg and to hepatitis B core antigen, resulting in ineffective cytotoxic T cell lysis of infected hepatocytes (**Chen et al., 2005**).

Phase 2

HBeAg-Positive Chronic Hepatitis

As the host immune system matures and begins to recognize HBV-related epitopes on hepatocytes, immune-mediated hepatocellular injury ensues. Although HBV replication continues in the liver and viremia is continual, the viral level in the serum becomes lower than during the immune tolerance phase when viral replication is completely unopposed (**Tedder *et al.*, 2002**). In patients with perinatally acquired HBV infection, transition from the immune tolerance to the HBeAg-positive chronic hepatitis phase occurs during the second or third decade of life.46 This phase is characterized by the presence of HBeAg, high levels of serum HBV DNA, elevation of serum aminotransferase levels, and histological findings of active inflammation and often fibrosis in the liver. Most patients with HBeAg-positive chronic hepatitis remain asymptomatic, making it difficult to detect the transition from the immune tolerance phase based on clinical grounds alone. However, some patients present with a symptomatic flare of hepatitis that mimics acute hepatitis or even with fulminant hepatic failure. These flares may precede the disappearance of HBeAg and the development of antibody against it, culminating in remission of hepatitis activity. However, some flares result in only transient decreases in serum HBV DNA levels without the clearance of HBeAg.32 Occasionally, hepatic decompensation may occur after these flares.

Spontaneous HBeAg seroconversion, which occurs annually in as many as 10% to 20% of those with HBeAg positive hepatitis, is an important landmark in the natural history of chronic HBV infection (**Yim and Lok, 2006**).

Factors associated with a higher rate of spontaneous HBeAg seroconversion include older age, higher aminotransferase levels (**Liaw, 2003**), and certain HBV genotypes (**Kao *et al.*, 2004**). High aminotransferase levels are considered surrogate markers for a vigorous host immune response that results in higher spontaneous and treatment-induced HBeAg seroconversion. In contrast, spontaneous HBeAg clearance or seroconversion occurs in fewer than 5% of patients with normal or mildly elevated levels of alanine aminotransferase (ALT) (**Yim and Lok, 2006**). Recent reports from Asian countries have shown that HBV genotype B, compared with genotype C, is associated with HBeAg seroconversion at an earlier age and with more sustained viral and biochemical remission after HBeAg seroconversion, resulting in a lower prevalence of HBeAg (**Kao *et al.*, 2004**). Many HBeAg-positive persons undergo seroconversion over time. However, those who remain HBeAg positive continue to be at risk for progressive liver disease. Approximately 12% to 20% of them will develop serious liver injury that results in cirrhosis and complications within 5 years, depending on the duration of the chronic hepatitis and the frequency and severity of flares (**McMahon *et al.*, 2001**).

Phase 3
Inactive HBsAg Carriers

After seroconversion, most patients remain negative for HBeAg and positive for anti-HBe antibody. Seroconversion is usually accompanied by stabilization of hepatitis, characterized by normalization of ALT levels and decreases in HBV DNA to low (<1000 copies/mL) or undetectable levels, depending on the assays used. This condition is commonly referred to as the "inactive carrier state."**Lok *et al.*, (2001)** Histologically, minimal to mild hepatitis may be observed, although the degree of fibrosis may be variable. For example, inactive cirrhosis may be identified in patients who had severe liver injury before seroconversion (**Yim and Lok, 2006**).

HBeAg reversion occurs in a minority of patients who have seroconversion. In a study by **McMahon, (2004)** 432 of 541 seroconverters (80%) remained HBeAg negative and anti-HBe positive throughout the study, whereas the other 109 (20%) seroreverted after the initial seroconversion. Seroreverting patients tended to fluctuate between seroconversion and seroreversion, commonly having 2 to 3 reversions over the 6 to 7 years of this study. Seroreversion episodes are frequently accompanied by a flare of hepatitis activity (**Perrillo, 2001**). In the study by **Hsu *et al.*, (2002)** 12 patients reverted to HBeAg positivity, 5 of whom developed cirrhosis during follow-

31

up. In addition to these spontaneous seroreversion episodes, HBV replication can reactivate in inactive HBV carriers as a result of immunosuppression or chemotherapy.

Spontaneous clearance of HBsAg was delayed in a small number of inactive HBV carriers, at the estimated annual rate of 0.5% to 2% in Western countries and at a much lower rate of 0.1% to 0.8% in Asian countries **(Yuen *et al.*, 2004)**.

Phase 4

HBeAg-Negative Chronic Hepatitis

Chronic hepatitis may recur in up to one third of inactive HBV carriers without reversion of HBeAg in their serum **(Funk *et al.*, 2002)**. Some of these carriers are likely infected with 1 of the HBV variants that cannot express HBeAg because of mutations in the precore or core-promoter regions of the HBV genome **(Chu *et al.*, 2003)**. Most patients progress to this phase after a variable length of time in the inactive HBV carrier state, whereas some progress to HBeAg-negative chronic hepatitis directly from HBeAg-positive chronic hepatitis **(Hsu *et al.*, 2002)**.

This phase is characterized by the absence of HBeAg, the presence of anti-HBe antibody, detectable levels of HBV DNA, elevated levels of serum ALT, and histological findings of continued necroinflammation of the liver. Compared to those with HBeAg-positive chronic hepatitis, patients with HBeAg-negative chronic hepatitis are generally older, have more advanced disease as evidenced by liver histology, and have lower serum HBV DNA levels **(Yim and Lok, 2006)**.

HBV Diagnosis

Various tests are used to diagnose hepatitis B and to assess the stage of disease and the extent of liver damage **(Franciscus** and **Highleyman, 2008)**.

> **Antibody Tests**

Hepatitis B is diagnosed and staged by looking at a complex combination of HBV antigens and antibodies. Tests are available to measure three HBV-associated proteins or antigens: HBsAg (surface), HBcAg (core), and HBeAg. The immune system produces three corresponding antibodies: called anti-HBs, anti-HBc, and anti-HBe. The presence of HBsAg and/or HBV DNA in the blood indicates that a person currently has hepatitis B. The presence of anti-HBs antibodies when HBsAg is absent shows that a person does not have active disease. People who have been exposed to HBV and have successfully cleared the infection test positive for both anti-HBs and anti-HBc. People who have received the HBV vaccine have anti-HBs but not anti-HBc. The presence of HBeAg often indicates that the virus is actively replicating and that a person is highly infectious and at greater risk for liver damage. Traditionally, the loss of HBeAg has been used as an indication that treatment is effective. However, when people have had HB for many years, they may test negative for HBeAg, but still have an active infection and high viral load. This is called HBeAg-negative hepatitis B. These cases result when HBV mutate and are able to replicate without HBeAg.

> **Serological Markers**

Hepatitis B surface antigen (HBsAg):

A protein on the surface of HBV; it can be detected in serum (blood) during acute or chronic HBV infection. The presence of HBsAg indicates a person is infectious. The body normally produces antibodies to HBsAg (anti-HBs) as part of its immune response to fight the infection. HBsAg is the antigen used to make hepatitis B vaccine.

Hepatitis B surface antibody (anti-HBs):

The presence of anti-HBs is generally interpreted as indicating recovery and immunity from HBV infection. Anti-HBs also develop in people who have been successfully vaccinated against hepatitis B.

Total hepatitis B core antibody (anti-HBc):

Positivity indicates a recent or current infection with HBV (≤ 6 months).

Hepatitis B "e" antigen (HBeAg):

This antigen, which can make up part of the virus's core, is found in serum during acute and chronic HB. Its presence can indicate that the virus is replicating rapidly and that the person has high levels of HBV. However, it is possible to be infected and have a high viral load if this antigen is absent. This can happen in adults who have had HB infection for many years. This is called HBeAg-negative HB.

Hepatitis B "e" antibody (HBeAb or anti-HBe):

This antibody is produced by the immune system during acute HBV infection or during active viral replication. Spontaneous conversion from HBeAg to anti-HBe (known as seroconversion) can indicate lower viral load in patients undergoing antiviral or interferon treatment. *adapted from *http://www.cdc.gov/NCIDOF/DISEASES/hepatitis/b/faqb.htm*

➢ **Viral Load Tests**

Viral load tests measure the amount of HBV DNA (genetic material) circulating in the blood. A detectable viral load indicates that HBV is actively replicating. In people with abnormal liver enzyme levels, higher HBV DNA viral load appears to be associated with more severe liver disease. Viral load tests are also useful as an indication of how well antiviral treatment is working.

➢ **Biochemical Tests**

Biochemical liver tests are a rough indication of the degree of liver inflammation. A hepatic panel includes measurements of various substances in the blood. Many – but not all – people with acute or chronic HB develop elevated levels of two liver enzymes called alanine aminotransferase (ALT, formerly known as SPGT) and aspartate aminotransferase (AST, formerly known as SGOT). ALT and AST are released into the blood when the liver is damaged. Elevated liver enzyme levels are often the first sign of liver problems, and a decrease in ALT often indicates that treatment is working. However, many people with hepatitis B have persistently normal liver enzyme levels. In addition, some people have normal ALT levels even though they have background cirrhosis.

Another common measure is bilirubin level. Bilirubin is a pigment that is continuously produced as a byproduct of the natural breakdown of red blood cells. Bilirubin level indicates the degree of liver function, as do serum albumin level and measures of blood clotting (**Franciscus** and **Highleyman, 2008**).

Because test results can vary from lab to lab, it is recommended that the same laboratory be used each time so that results can be compared. Keep copies of your lab results for future reference.

> ➢ **Genotype Tests**

HBV has several different genotypes or strains, lettered A through H. Different HBV genotypes are associated with varying levels of viral replication, liver disease progression, and treatment success. In the United States, the following genotypes are commonly found: genotype A (35%), genotype B (22%), genotype C (31%), genotype D (10%). HBV genotype testing is becoming more common because some genotypes respond better to certain drugs than others. For example, genotypes A and B may respond better to interferon treatment than genotypes C and D. Researchers are also finding that viral mutations, or risk of liver damage, may depend on the type of genotype.

> ➢ **Liver Biopsy**

Biopsies are done to assess the extent of inflammation and the amount of scarring of the liver. Biopsy is the most reliable indicator of liver damage and is used to help make decisions about treatment. Many doctors do not recommend biopsies for HBV carriers with normal biochemical liver tests. In the most common biopsy procedure, the abdominal skin and muscle are numbed and a long, thin needle is quickly inserted into the liver to draw out a small sample of tissue, which is examined under a microscope. Complications from liver biopsies are rare. If you are anxious about the procedure, ask your doctor for a mild tranquilizer prior to the biopsy and for pain medication afterwards.

HBV Treatment

There are currently two types of drug treatments for chronic HB: interferon and antivirals. Research suggests that one day combination or sequential treatment may be used effectively against hepatitis B. HB treatment is more likely to be beneficial if a person has elevated liver enzymes (ALT), and low viral load. Treatment for people with very low HBV DNA levels and normal ALT levels is not usually recommended because this shows there is no liver damage occurring. A majority of people chronically infected with HBV will never require treatment, but should have their ALT levels and overall health monitored regularly at least every six months **(Franciscus** and **Highleyman, 2008)**.

> **Approved Treatments**

alfa-2a, Pegasys, a genetically engineered product based on natural immune system proteins. Pegylation is a process by which polyethylene glycol is attached to standard interferon in order to prolong its activity in the body so fewer HBV can escape its effects. This interferon drug that is produced by Roche requires one weekly injection over 48 weeks. This interferon has replaced conventional interferon (interferon-alpha 2b), which was less effective and required three weekly injections. In clinical trials, about 25 to 35 percent of people with HBeAg-positive HB were able to clear the HBeAg and develop the "e" antibody after treatment with pegylated interferon.

Pegylated interferon appears to be more successful in HBeAg-positive patients with genotypes A and B. Studies also show that people with HBeAg-negative hepatitis B, who also have elevated ALTs and detectable viral load, also benefit from pegylated interferon. About 63 percent experienced lowered viral load with pegylated interferon and about 38 percent achieved normal ALT levels. Because interferon stimulates the body's immune response, interferon can temporarily worsen liver inflammation (a "flare"). Most experts recommend that people with decompensated cirrhosis should not be treated with interferon. Pegylated interferon has not yet been approved for children with HB.

Warning: **In March of 2008,** *both the Eurpean Health Agency (CHMP) and Health Canada issued a warning about combining interferon with Telbivudine (Sebivo, Tyzeka) because of the risk of peripheral neuropathy* **(Franciscus** and **Highleyman, 2008**).

> ➤ **Antivirals:**

Lamivudine (Epivir-HBV) is an antiviral drug that inhibits HBV replication. The drug is typically taken daily for at least 48 weeks and produces undetectable HBV DNA and normal ALTs in 40 percent of cases. Unfortunately, lamivudine treatment leads to the development of lamivudine-resistant HBV mutants at a rate of 10–27 percent after one year, 37–48 percent after two years, and 60–65 percent after four years of treatment. Once a patient has developed viral resistance to lamivudine, he or she may also develop resistance to similar antivirals. This is the only antiviral approved by the FDA for treatment of children.

Adefovir (Hepsera) produces substantial decreases in HBV DNA viral load (21 percent in HBeAg-positive people and 51 percent in HBeAg-negtive people), reductions in ALT level, and lessening of liver damage if a patient has not been treated with any other antiviral. Adefovir appears to work well against both wild or non-mutated HBV and lamivudine-resistant HBV as long as adefovir is added to ongoing lamivudine treatment. The drug is associated with kidney toxicity in some people.

Entecavir (Baraclude) is another antiviral that works best when patients have never been treated with an antiviral (called treatment naïve). In HBeAg-positive patients, entecavir reduces viral load in 67 percent of people, leads to HBeAg seroconverion (production of the "e" antibody) in 21 percent, and produces normal ALTs in 68 percent. In the HBeAg-negative, it produces undetectable HBV DNA in 90 percent and normal ALTs in 78 percent. Entecavir resistance remains under 1 percent after one year in treatment-naïve patients. However, in patients who have already developed lamivudine resistance, entecavir resistance reaches 43% after just four years.

Telbivudine (Tyzeka), produces undetectable HBV DNA in 60 percent of HBeAg-positive, treatment-naïve patients, an HBeAg seroconversion rate of 26 percent, and a normal ALT rate of 77 percent. In HBeAg-negative, treatment-naïve patients, telbivudine produces undetectable HBV DNA rates in 88 percent and normal ALT rates in 74 percent. It has a resistance rate of 3-4 percent after one year and 9-22 percent after two years. While the U.S. FDA has not approved combination treatment with pegylated interferon and an antiviral, some physicians are experimenting with combined or sequential treatment using these two drugs.

Warning: *Recently, Canada's drug safety commission issued a warning against taking the antiviral telbivudine (brand name Tyzeka in the U.S. and Sebivo in Canada) with interferon. Ten percent of patients treated with the drug combination developed peripheral neuropathy– weakness, numbness, tingling and burning sensations in the arms and/or legs – about three months after treatment began.*

Tenofovir (Viread) the newest antiviral was approved by **the FDA in August 2008**. It has been used successfully against HIV for years. Viread (tenofovir disoproxil fumarate) is a nucleotide analog reverse transcriptase and HBV polymerase inhibitor that blocks an enzyme that the hepatitis B virus needs to replicate in liver cells. The recommended dose for chronic hepatitis B is one 300-mg tablet a day. Two ongoing Phase III clinical trials comparing Viread with Hepsera found that chronic hepatitis B patients on Viread achieved a higher rate of complete treatment response compared with patients taking Hepsera, according to the company, which says the two drugs should not be used together.

➢ **Alternative Therapies**

In addition to pharmaceutical drugs, some people use alternative and complementary therapies for hepatitis B. Herbs often used for chronic hepatitis include milk thistle (silymarin), licorice root (glycyrrhizin), and phyllanthus. Herbal remedies should be treated like drugs, since they may have side effects and can interact with other herbs and conventional medications. Many herbs can be toxic to the liver, including chaparral, germander, kava kava, and plants that contain pyrrolizidine alkaloids. (Herbal therapies are discussed in more detail in a separate fact sheet from the Hepatitis C Support Project: See the section Hepatitis C and Complementary and Alternative Medicine (CAM) at *http://www.hcvadvocate.org/hepatitis/factsheets.asp.*) Nutritional supplements suggested for hepatitis B include vitamin C, vitamin E, glutathione, N-acetyl-cysteine, S-adenosylmethionine (SAM-e), and thymic factors. Make sure to contact a reputable herbalist or nutritionist and inform all your health-care providers about any herbs, supplements, or other alternative therapies you are using.

➢ **Clinical Trials**

The process of testing a new drug involves establishing its safety and toxicity in humans (Phase I trials), measuring its safety and tolerability (Phase II trials), and comparing the new drug to current standard treatments or placebo (Phase III trials). After the FDA has granted approval and the new drug is marketed, ongoing studies are done to refine the treatment for maximum safety and effectiveness (Phase IV, or post-marketing trials). Clinical trials can be a good way to obtain free medication; some trials also may cover the costs of laboratory tests (although they may not provide the results to you or your doctor). Be aware that clinical trial participants typically are randomized to receive either the experimental drug or a standard treatment or placebo (an inactive substance used as a control); you may not be chosen to receive the new drug or the most effective dosage. Read all the clinical trial information and make sure that you fully understand the terms and conditions before you give your informed consent to participate.

➢ **Nucleic acid-based Antiviral Approaches to HBV**

Nucleic acid-based approaches are actively being pursued as antiviral therapy for chronic HBV infection. The therapeutic potential of ribozymes, antisense molecules, dominant negative mutant proteins, intracellular antibodies and DNA-based vaccination. has been clearly demonstrated in experimental systems both *in vitro* and *in vivo*. Future studies will need to evaluate these antiviral strategies in established or new animal systems involving ducks, woodchucks, and nude or transgenic mice. More effective methods of targeted gene delivery systems to all infected hepatocytes will have to be developed. It may also be necessary to pursue regulated gene expression systems for optimal therapeutic results. Due to genetic mutations, escape of HBV from nucleic acid-based strategies is anticipated and viral resistance may occur. Preclinical trials of pharmacokinetic, pharmacodynamic and toxic profiles of these new molecular agents will be required to ensure a safe translation to human subjects. Under these conditions, nucleic acid-based antiviral strategies may eventually contribute to existing therapies and augment the treatment and prevention of chronic HBV infection (**Spangenberg and Wands, 2003**).

HBV viral DNA is transcribed in several viral RNAs, and serves as the template for translation into viral proteins. HBV pregenomic RNA is reverse transcribed into viral DNA. Ribozymes, ODN and antisense RNA may bind to and interfere with viral RNA. Dominant negative mutants and intracellular antibodies may interfere with viral proteins. The host immune response against viral proteins may be augmented by DNA-based immunization (**Figure 10**).

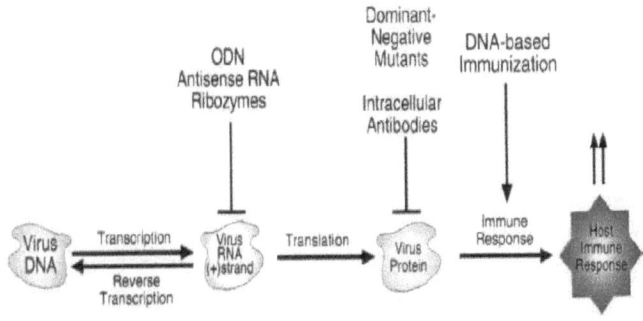

Figure (10). Steps in the viral life cycle of HBV and potential targets of nucleic acid-based approaches to HBV.

➤ Managing Drug Side Effects

Drugs used to treat HBV are often associated with side effects. Common side effects of interferon include flulike symptoms, fatigue, nausea, diarrhea, headache, muscle and joint aches, depression, and anxiety; less common side effects include hair loss and thyroid dysfunction. Side effects of antivirals are uncommon, but may include nausea, diarrhea, and headache; rarer side effects include low blood cell counts, peripheral neuropathy (nerve damage in the hands and feet), and pancreatitis (inflammation of the pancreas). Some physical symptoms may be reduced with lowdose ibuprofen (do not take if you have cirrhosis) or acetaminophen (high doses can be toxic to the liver). People experiencing psychological symptoms such as depression, anxiety, or irritability may find antidepressants helpful. Some people find that injecting interferon just before bedtime lets them sleep through the worst side effects. Vary where you inject your interferon to prevent skin irritation or a rash at the injection site. To manage gastrointestinal symptoms, eat small, frequent healthy meals or snacks rather than three large meals each day, and avoid spicy or fatty foods. Many people find that side effects are worse when they first start taking a new drug but diminish over time. Talk to your health-care provider about other ways to manage treatment side effects, and inform him or her if your symptoms get worse.

HBV Management

Chronic HB can be a difficult disease to manage. However, there are steps you can take to cope with the disease and keep your liver as healthy as possible. People infected with HB should receive regular medical attention. Biochemical liver tests should be monitored regularly (every 6-12 months). During treatment, levels of HBV DNA also should be measured to gauge how well therapy is working. People taking interferon should be monitored for side effects, including blood cell counts, thyroid function tests, and assessment of depression. People with inactive HBV should receive regular ALT tests. All HBV carriers should be screened for liver cancer. It is important to find a doctor who is knowledgeable about HB; hepatologists and gastroenterologists specialize in liver disease. If you are not comfortable with your doctor, ask family or friends to recommend someone they like.

HBV Prevention Guidelines

- Get vaccinated against HB.
- Infants born to HBV-infected mothers should receive the HB vaccine and HBV immune globulin (HBIG) on the day of birth.
- Practice safer sex, including the use of latex condoms and barriers.
- Do not share needles to inject drugs; obtain new needles from a needle exchange or – if you must share – clean needles thoroughly with bleach
- Do not share drug equipment such as cocaine straws or crack pipes.
- Tattooists, piercers, and acupuncturists should use new needles for each client.
- Manicurists and barbers should disinfect tools between customers or use disposable, single-use items.
- Do not share personal items such as razors, toothbrushes, nail files, or pierced earrings.
- Exercise universal precautions in health-care settings, including the use of latex gloves.
- Properly dispose of used needles, bandages, and menstrual supplies; clean and disinfect spilled body fluids.
- Cover all cuts, sores, and rashes.

> ***Healthy Liver Tips***

- Get regular health check-ups, including biochemical liver tests.
- Avoid or limit consumption of alcohol and recreational drugs.
- Take no more than the recommended doses of medications.
- Be careful when using multiple drugs, herbs, or drugs and herbs together.
- Eat a healthy, well-balanced diet.
- Get regular, moderate exercise.
- Inform all your health-care providers about all drugs, herbs, supplements, and alternative therapies you are using.

- Inform all your doctors and other health-care providers about your HB, especially if you need cancer treatment or steroid therapy.

> **Nutrition**

Because the liver processes everything you eat and drink, a healthy, well-balanced diet is important. A healthy diet should follow the general guidelines based on the new Food Guide Pyramid – *www.mypyramid.gov*. Such a diet is low in fat and sodium, high in complex carbohydrates, and has adequate protein. Today, dietary restrictions do not play a major role in managing chronic HB. Processed foods often contain chemical additives, so reduce consumption of canned, frozen, and other preserved foods. Eat organic fruits and vegetables to avoid pesticides and fertilizers. Read labels and become familiar with ingredients. Many doctors recommend that people with hepatitis avoid raw or undercooked shellfish such as oysters and clams, because they may contain infectious organisms or toxins. A well-balanced diet should contain all essential vitamins and minerals; avoid taking high-dose supplements – especially those containing vitamin A, vitamin D, or iron, which can be harmful to the liver. Consult a licensed dietitian for specific dietary recommendations and seek medical advice before undertaking any unconventional diet.

> **Alcohol, Drugs, and Toxins**

People with HB – especially those with cirrhosis should avoid consuming excessive amounts of alcohol.

Certain drugs – prescription, over-the-counter, and recreational – and herbal remedies can be harmful to the liver (hepatotoxic), especially when taken in high doses or used in combination. People with HBV should inform their health-care providers about all drugs, herbal remedies, and supplements they are taking. Avoid or reduce consumption of recreational drugs. Do not exceed recommended drug doses. Because the liver processes toxins, avoid exposure to toxic liquids and fumes such as solvents, paint thinners, pesticides, and aerosol sprays. If it is necessary to use such chemicals, work in a well-ventilated area, cover your skin, and wear gloves and a protective face mask (**Franciscus** and **Highleyman, 2008**).

> **General Wellness**

Exercise:

Regular aerobic exercise can improve overall fitness and may help reduce fatigue, stress, and depression. Most people with chronic hepatitis can safely engage in moderate exercise. Avoid exercise if you are feeling very ill. People with advanced cirrhosis should be cautious about lifting weights. All people with chronic hepatitis should consult their health-care provider before starting an exercise program.

Stress management:

Controlling stress is a major factor in managing any chronic disease. Exercise, meditation, and time management can all help reduce stress. Try to maintain a realistic picture of your health and a positive attitude.

Managing fatigue:

Fatigue and low energy levels are reported by some people with HBV. Learn your limits and try not to overextend yourself. Take naps as needed and get enough sleep at night. Remember that your health is important; learn to say "no" to friends and family who have unrealistic expectations of your energy level.

Time management:

Plan activities in advance and try to make realistic work and play schedules. Many people find it helpful to use a daily planner to help schedule and remember activities. Don't forget to plan restful activities.

Meditation:

Many people find meditation (a method of relaxation and clearing and focusing the mind) to be a useful tool in coping with chronic hepatitis. Meditation can reduce stress and help you maintain a healthy outlook on life. There are many meditation traditions, some of which are simple and easy to learn **(Franciscus** and **Highleyman, 2008)**.

➢ Support Groups and Therapy

Many people with HB feel isolated and find it difficult to cope with the effects of living with a chronic illness. A support group can offer a safe space to discuss the emotional issues surrounding chronic hepatitis. In addition, information shared by peers can be helpful in making decisions, managing symptoms, and developing coping strategies. Some people also find therapy with a psychologist or social worker to be beneficial **(Franciscus** and **Highleyman, 2008)**.

National HB Strategies

We Need HB Strategies in our countries:

Strategy 1: Improve **HBV**-related Public Health Prevention Infrastructure

Strategy 2: Increase **HBV**-related Health Education and Awareness

Strategy 3: Increase Screenings for Chronic **HBV** Infection

Strategy 4: Improve Access to Care and Treatment for Chronic **HBV**

Strategy 5: Increase **Research** for **HBV** and Liver Cancer

Partnerships:

- Ministries of Health &Population
- Ministries of High Education and Scientific Research
- Privet Sectors
- World Health Organization (WHO

Goal: Reduce the risk of chronic hepatitis B virus (**HBV**) infection and its long-term complications

Objectives:

• Prevent new **HBV** infections by promoting screening, immunization and education

• Promote early detection, appropriate follow-up and clinical management of persons with chronic **HBV** infection

• Increase awareness and support of **HBV research.**

Indicators:

1. Reduce the number of notifications of new cases of HB infection in line with the National Healthcare Agreement indicator.

2. Improve the health and wellbeing of people with chronic hepatitis B, through access to clinical services, treatment, education and support.

3. Reduce hepatitis B-related stigma and discrimination.

4. Incorporate hepatitis B-related prevention and treatment into broader health reforms.

Research & Surveillance

Research is critical to providing the evidence base for the development and implementation of policies and programs at all levels of the national response to chronic hepatitis B.

Limited data are available describing the impact of chronic hepatitis B, and how the communities most affected by the condition respond to this infection. The evidence base for an effective public health response to the hepatitis B epidemic will be established through well-conducted national and international research. Acute and chronic hepatitis B infection cases are routinely notified through public health surveillance systems with limited demographic information.

Priority actions in research and surveillance

· Develop a national hepatitis B surveillance strategy, under the supervision of all partners.

Conclusion

While HB can have serious consequences, most people infected with HBV do not develop chronic disease and lead normal lives. Inactive carriers show evidence of HBV infection but do not have symptoms of liver dysfunction. A minority of people chronically infected with HBV develop progressive disease that can lead to serious liver damage, including cirrhosis, liver cancer, and liver failure. New drugs for HBV are being developed. Universal HBV vaccination presents the best hope for controlling the spread of HB. Beyond medical treatment, if you have HBV there are several steps you can take – including getting regular medical care, avoiding alcohol and drugs, eating a healthy diet, engaging in moderate exercise, managing stress and fatigue, and joining a support group – to keep your liver as healthy as possible and to improve your overall quality of life.

The dynamic balance between viral replication and host immune response plays a key role in the pathogenesis of liver disease from HBV infection. Most infections in immunocompetent adults are resolved, whereas most neonates and infants develop chronic HBV infection. Those with chronic HBV infection may present in 1 of 4 phases. Of these, the HBeAg-positive and -negative chronic hepatitis phases are associated with a significant risk of progression to cirrhosis. Several risk factors such as HBV DNA levels, HBeAg status, and ALT levels have been identified to predict long-term outcome such as cirrhosis and HCC. These data highlight the importance of monitoring all patients with chronic HBV infection to identify treatment candidates and select optimal timing for treatment, to recognize those at risk for complications, and to implement surveillance for HCC.

It is still essential to prevent the spread of wild, vaccine-sensitive strains of HBV. Well-tested measures such as safe sex and avoiding the risks associated with injection drug use will also help to reduce horizontal transmission of both the wild virus and VEMs. HB immunization for infants of mothers with HBV will reduce perinatal transmission of the wild virus but may not prevent transmission of VEMs.

The global hepatitis B immunization programme will continue to reduce new incident infections of hepatitis B and the burden of chronic HBV disease globally, although it is simultaneously generating VEMs. One simulation has predicted that the spread of VEMs selected out by immunization would result in relatively few new infections for the foreseeable future. However, it is not yet clear whether the emergence of ADAP-VEMs in a population will be speeded up by the simultaneous use of both the vaccine and treatment. Of course, hepatitis B vaccines that incorporate HBV proteins not altered by immunization or drug therapy are the ultimate solution to prevent the appearance of viral escape mutants generated by vaccines or antiviral drugs.

References

Remember that not all the information you find on the Internet is correct. The Internet contains a wealth of information – both good and bad. Always check the **sources** *of the information you find online. Look for* **dates** *and* **references**.

> **Research & Review Articles**

Ali BA; Huang TH and Xie, QD (**2005**): Detection and Expression of Hepatitis B Virus X Gene in One and Two-Cell Embryos from Golden Hamster Oocytes in Vitro Fertilized with Human Spermatozoa Carrying HBV DNA. *Molecular Reproduction and Development 70: 30-36. Published online December 2004.*

Ali BA; Huang, TH; Salem HH *et al.,* (**2006a**): Expression of hepatitis B virus genes in early embryonic cells originated from hamster ova and human spermatozoa transfected with the complete viral genome. *Asian Journal of Andrology 8:273-279.*

Ali BA; Salem HH; Huang TH *et al.,* (**2006b**): Detection of full length HB S gene (1.2 kb) in one- and two-cell embryo originated from hamster oocyte and human spermatozoa by using nested-PCR. *Journal of Medical Sciences 6: 1015-1020.*

Ali BA; Salem HH; Wang XM *et al.,* (**2009**): Detection of hepatitis B polymerase gene in early embryonic cells from golden hamster oocyte and human spermatozoa carrying HBV DNA. *International Journal of Virology 5:* 164-169.

Arankalle VA; Murhekar KM; Gandhe SS *et al.,* (**2003**). Hepatitis B virus: predominance of genotype D in primitive tribes of the Andaman and Nicobar islands, India (1989–1999). *J Gen Virol 84:1915–1920.*

Arauz-Ruiz P; NorderH; Robertson BH *et al.,* (**2002**). Genotype H: A new Amerindian genotype of hepatitis B virus revealed in Central America. *J Gen Virol 83:2059–2073.*

Chen M; Sallberg M; Hughes J *et al.,* (**2005**). Immune tolerance split between hepatitis B virus precore and core proteins. *J Virol. 79:3016-3027.*

Chu CJ; Keeffe EB; Han SH *et al.,* **(2003)**. US HBV Epidemiology Study Group. Prevalence of HBV precore/core promoter variants in the United States. *Hepatology.* 38:619-628.

Clements CJ; Coghlan B; Creati M *et al.,* **(2010)**. Global control of hepatitis B virus: does treatment-induced antigenic change affect immunization?. *Bulletin of the World Health Organization* 88:66-73.

Divi RL; Leonard SL; Kuo MM *et al.,* **(2005)**. Cardiac mitochondrial compromise in 1-yr-old Erythrocebus patas monkeys perinatally-exposed to nucleoside reverse transcriptase inhibitors. *Cardiovasc Toxicol 5: 333-346.*

Funk ML; Rosenberg DM and Lok AS **(2002)**. World-wide epidemiology of HBeAg-negative chronic hepatitis B and associated precore and core promoter variants. *J Viral Hepatology.* 9:52-61.

Gandhe SS; Chadha MS and Arankalle VA **(2003)**. Hepatitis B virus genotypes and serotypes in western India: lack of clinical significance. *J Med Virol 69:324–330.*

Hsu YS; Chien RN; Yeh CT *et al.,* **(2002)**. Long-term outcome after spontaneous HBeAg seroconversion in patients with chronic hepatitis B. *Hepatology.* 35:1522-1527.

Idrees M; Khan S and Riazuddin S **(2004)**. Common genotypes of hepatitis B virus. *J Coll Physicians Surg Pak 14:44–47.*

Kao JH; Chen PJ; Lai MY *et al.,* **(2000)**. Hepatitis B genotypes correlate with clinical outcomes in patients with chronic hepatitis B. *Gastroenterology 118:54–59.*

Kao JH; Chen PJ; Lai MY *et al.,* **(2004)**. Hepatitis B virus genotypes and spontaneous hepatitis B e antigen seroconversion in Taiwanese hepatitis B carriers. *J Med Virol.* 72:363-369.

Kazim SN; Wakil SM; Khan LA *et al.,* **(2002)**. Vertical transmission of hepatitis B virus despite maternal lamivudine therapy. *Lancet 359: 1488-1489.*

Lee C; Gong Y; Brok J *et al., (2006)*. Effect of hepatitis B immunisation in newborn infants of mothers positive for hepatitis B surface antigen: systematic review and meta-analysis. *BMJ 332: 328-336.*

Liaw YF **(2003)**. Hepatitis flares and hepatitis B e antigen seroconversion: implication in anti-hepatitis B virus therapy. *J Gastroenterol Hepatol*18: 246-252.

Liaw YF; Leung N; Kao JH *et al.*, **(2008)**. Asian-Pacific consensus statement of the management of chronic hepatitis B: a 2008 update. Hepatology International 2008.

Lok AS; Heathcote EJ; Hoofnagle JH **(2001)**. Management of hepatitis B: 2000— summary of a workshop. *Gastroenterology*. 120:1828-1853.

Lok AS and McMahon BJ **(2007)**. Chronic hepatitis B. *Hepatology* 45: 507-539

Mast EE; Margolis HS; Fiore AE *et al.*, **(2005)**. A comprehensive immunization strategy to eliminate transmission of hepatitis B virus infection in the United States: recommendations of the Advisory Committee on Immunization Practices (ACIP) part 1: immunization of infants, children, and adolescents. *MMWR Recomm Rep 54: 1-31.*

McMahon BJ **(2004)**. The natural history of chronic hepatitis B virus infection. *Semin Liver Dis.* 24:17-21.

McMahon BJ; Holck P; Bulkow L *et al.*, **(2001)**. Serologic and clinical outcomes of 1536 Alaska Natives chronically infected with hepatitis B virus. *Ann Intern Med.* 135:759-768.

Mogahed FAK **(2009)**. Molecular study on the genome of hepatitis B virus (HBV). *M.Sc thesis, Faculty of Science, Alexandria University.*

Orito E; Ichida T; Sakugawa H *et al.*, **(2001a)**. Geographic distribution of hepatitis B virus (HBV) genotype in patients with chronic HBV in Japan. *Hepatology 34:590–594.*

Orito E; Mizokami M; Sakugawa H *et al.*, **(2001b)**. A control study for clinical and molecular differences between hepatitis B viruses of genotypes B and C. *Hepatology 33:218–233.*

Perrillo RP **(2001)**. Acute flares in chronic hepatitis B: the natural and unnatural history of an immunologically mediated liver disease. *Gastroenterology*. 120:1009-1022.

Pungpapong S; Kim WR and Poterucha JJ **(2007)**. Natural History of Hepatitis B Virus Infection: An Update for Clinicians. *Mayo Clin Proc. 82:967-975.*

Sakurai M; Sugauchi F; Suzuki S *et al.,* **(2004)**. Genotype and phylogenetic characterization of hepatitis B virus among ethnic cohort in Hawaii. *World J.gastroenterol 10: 2218–2222.*

Saudy N; Sugauchi F; Tanaka Y *et al.,* **(2003)**. Genotypes and phylogenetic characterization of hepatitis B and delta viruses in Egypt. *J Med Virol 70:529-536.*

Soderstrom A; Norkrans G and Lindh M **(2003)**. Hepatitis B virus DNA during pregnancy and post partum: aspects on vertical transmission. *Scand J Infect Dis* 35: 814-819.

Sookoian S **(2006)**. Annals of Hepatology, Symposium on liver & pregnancy Effect of pregnancy on pre-existing liver disease:Chronic viral hepatitis. *Annals of Hepatology 5:190-197.*

Su GG; Pan KH; Zhao NF *et al.,* **(2004)**. Efficacy and safety of lamivudine treatment for chronic hepatitis B in pregnancy. *World J Gastroenterol 10: 910-912.*

Sugauchi F; Orito E; Ichida T *et al.,* **(2002)**. Hepatitis B virus of genotype B with or without recombination with genotype C over the pre-core plus the core gene. *J Virol 76: 5985–5992.*

Tajiri H; Miyoshi Y; Funada S *et al.,* **(2001)**. Prospective study of mother-to-infant transmission of hepatitis C virus. *Pediatr Infect Dis J* 20: 10-14.

Tedder RS; Ijaz S; Gilbert N *et al.,* **(2002)**. Evidence for a dynamic host-parasite relationship in e-negative hepatitis B carriers. *J Med Virol.* 68:505-512.

Thibault V; Aubron-Olivier C; Agut H *et al.,* **(2002)**. Primary infection with a lamivudine-resistant hepatitis B virus. *AIDS* 16: 131-133.

Wang JS; Zhu QR and Wang XH **(2003)**. Breastfeeding does not pose any additional risk of immunoprophylaxis failure on infants of HBV carrier mothers. *Int J Clin Pract* 57: 100-102.

Xu DZ; Yan YP; Choi BC *et al.,* **(2002)**. Risk factors and mechanism of transplacental transmission of hepatitis B virus: a case-control study. *J Med Virol 67: 20-26.*

Yim HJ and Lok AS **(2006)**. Natural history of chronic hepatitis B virus infection: what we knew in 1981 and what we know in 2005. *Hepatology* 43:173-181.

Yuen MF; Wong DK; Sablon E *et al.,* **(2004)**. HBsAg seroclearance in chronic hepatitis B in the Chinese: virological, histological, and clinical aspects. *Hepatology.* 39:1694-1701.

➢ **Links**

- CDC Hepatitis Branch home page: www.cdc.gov/ncidod/diseases/hepatitis Hepatitis B Foundation: 215-489-4900; www.hepb.org.

- American Liver Foundation Hepatitis and Liver Disease : www.liverfoundation.org

- Hepatitis Central: www.hepatitiscentral.com

- Hepatitis Foundation International: www.hepfi.org

- Hepatitis Information Network: www.hepnet.com

- HIV and Hepatitis: www.hivandhepatitis.com/

- American Academy of Microbiology. *The Scientific Future of DNA for Immunization.* 1996. http://www.asmusa.org/acasrc/Colloquia/dnareprt.pdf

- The Big Book of Viruses. http://www.virology.net/Big_Virology/BVHomePage.html

- Center for Disease Control. http://www.cdc.gov/ncidod/diseases/hepatitis/b/index.htm

- DNAvaccine.com http://dnavaccine.com/

- Hepatitis B. http://cpmcnet.columbia.edu/dept/gi/hepB.html

- Garces, Robert. The Hepatitis B Virus Page. http://www.globalserve.net/~harlequin/HBV/

- The Hepatitis B Virus Research Programme. http://hbvrp.wits.ac.za/index.htm

- Immunization Action Coalition.

http://www.immunize.org/images/ca.d/ipcd1861/img0022.htm

- *Vaccination*   *Home*   *Page*

http://www.micro.unsw.edu.au/MICR3051%202001/Sasson,%20Gately,%20Karikios/VACCINE%20HOME.htm

- HBV publications *www.hbvadvocate.org/hepatitis/factsheets.asp*
- *Bulletin of the World Health Organization*

https://www.who.int/bulletin/volumes/88/1/08-065722/en/print.html

> **Books**

- Hepatitis B Virus by **Sandra S. Chaves,** In: Explore Travel Health with the New 2010 Yellow Book!. The Yellow Book is published every two years by CDC as a reference for those who advise international travelers about health risks. The Yellow Book is written primarily for health professionals, but others find it very useful.

- Living with with Hepatitis B: A Survivor's Guide. By **Gregory T. Everson**, MD and **Hedy Weinberg**. Hatherleigh Press (800-528-2550).

- The First Year—Hepatitis B: An Essential Guide for the Newly Diagnosed. By **William Finley** Green. Marlowe & Company.

- A Basic Guide to Hepatitis B. Hepatitis C support Project. By **Alan Franciscus** and Liz Highleyman, Version 4.1 August 2008.

- Novel approaches in the management of chronic HB V infection, by **Bartholomeusz** A; P Furman and S Locarnini. In: *Frontiers in Viral Hepatitis Ed. by RF Schinazi, J-P Sommadossi and CM Rice.* 225 — 243. (2003).

- The Molecular Biology of Hepatitis B Virus, by **TSB Yen**. In *Hepatitis Viruses*, ed. Ou, J.-H. James. Kluwer Academic Publishers, Norwell, Massachusetts, pp 51-79.

- Nucleic acid-based antiviral approaches to HBV. By **HC Spangenberg** and JR Wands.In: *Frontiers in Viral Hepatitis Ed. by RF Schinazi, J-P Sommadossi and CM Rice.* 139- 156. 2003

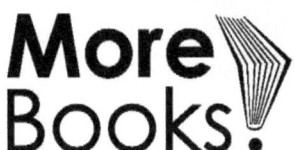
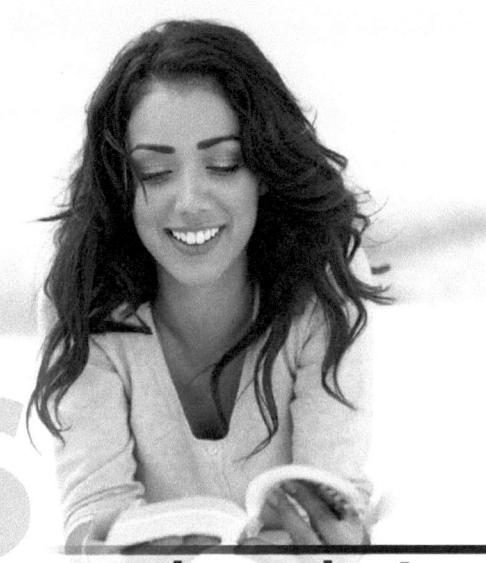
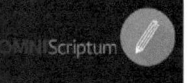

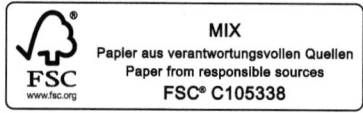